CONTENTS

FOREWORD   2

THE WORK OF FORESIGHT   3

THE FORESIGHT PROGRAMME   6

PART ONE — NUTRITION   9

PART TWO — HAIR ANALYSIS &
    SUPPLEMENT PROGRAMMES   14

  Mineral Deficiencies
  and Supplementation   18

PART THREE — HEALTH &

        LIFESTYLE ADVICE   22

  Alcohol, Tobacco and Street Drugs   22

  Genito-urinary and Other Infections 28

  Family Planning   30

  Allergies and Parasites   33

  Electromagnetic Radiation   35

  Other Hazards   36

SUMMARY   38

FORESIGHT PUBLICATIONS   39

CONTACTS   40

FOREWORD

Neal's Yard Remedies is delighted to be working with Foresight to provide you with information, help and advice, on overcoming infertility and planning for a healthy pregnancy and a healthy baby.

Foresight have developed a 3 part programme based on:
- Excellent nutrition and dietary advice
- Hair mineral analysis and individually tailored supplement programmes
- Lifestyle advice on dangers to avoid in the environment

Using the Foresight Programme, more than 70% of couples who have had problems conceiving go on to have healthy babies.

Neal's Yard Remedies therapists throughout the UK are trained by Foresight to give practical help and advice for couples trying to conceive.
- As part of the programme your therapist will take a hair sample and send to the Foresight laboratory for analysis to see if there are any nutritional problems or excess toxins in the system.
- An individual health and nutrition diet is then recommended to give couples the best chance of conceiving.
- Couples are then assessed for excess minerals or deficiencies and a supplement programme is recommended.
- Both partners are part of this process so that each member of the couple is in an optimum state of health and nutrition before trying for a baby.
- Follow up visits are recommended to assess and add supplements if required to assist in the development of conception.
- It may be that alternative therapies will be recommended as part of the process – for example, homœopathy, acupuncture, or reflexology, can help with specific issues.

When you visit one of our trained Foresight practitioners, they will be able to take your hair sample and guide you through the supplements programme. This will be in addition to nutritional and lifestyle advice and any other therapies that will help you.

We are delighted to support this booklet, to help you understand the essentials of the Foresight Programme and highlight some of the key factors that can affect fertility. We encourage you to find out more about the natural holistic approach that has been so successful helping thousands of couples to start a happy and healthy family.

To talk to one of our Foresight practitioners, ask at any Neal's Yard Remedies store throughout the UK, call our advice line 01747 834634 or contact Foresight on 01243 868001.

Susan Curtis, Registered Foresight Therapist
Medicines Director, Neal's Yard Remedies

THE WORK OF FORESIGHT

First established in 1978, Foresight is a charitable organisation networking worldwide with headquarters in West Sussex, England, whose primary role is to promote the importance of good health and nutritional status in both parents before conceiving a baby, and to provide information and advice on how the environment affects preconception health.

BENEFITS OF PRE-CONCEPTION CARE

Foresight has put together a thoroughly researched pre-conception programme which identifies and addresses various areas of concern in the health of prospective parents. The objective is to optimise the health of both prospective parents well before conception occurs so that a pregnancy can be started with normal, strong sperm and ovum and the embryo can implant and develop under optimum conditions in a healthy uterus, with no danger of damage from nutritional deficiency, toxins or disease.

Over the last twenty-nine years, Foresight has found that under these conditions it is possible to have uncomplicated pregnancies resulting in strong, healthy and perfectly formed babies, even in many couples who may have previously experienced the distress of infertility, miscarriage, stillbirth, birth defects, post-natal depression, health problems in the child, and other problems relating to conception, pregnancy and birth.

MODERN LIFE

It is a sad fact that the modern, busy lives that many people lead today, with our polluted air and our over-stored, over-processed and over-packaged foods, are not conducive to healthy living. Unfortunately, our ability to reproduce is one of the first things to be affected although of course the actual symptoms of 'sub-fertility' often do not become apparent until problems with conception or pregnancy result. Many couples experiencing reproductive problems of one form or another would otherwise consider themselves to be perfectly healthy.

Many thousands of much wanted babies are miscarried or stillborn each year, and many are born unnecessarily damaged or frail for want of all this vital information. It is so important to pass on this knowledge to help all parents to achieve a healthy, full term pregnancy.

In many, many cases, this can be achieved without resorting to "high tech", even where this has been recommended by the medics.

If a natural conception can be achieved, this negates the need for much travelling, stress, expense, invasive procedures and the use of hormonal drugs which are known to carry a cancer risk. The Department of Health states that Clomid should not be used for more than 3 months, and the GMC says a maximum of 6 cycles in any one woman's life-time. The effects on the babies have never been explored for the long-term. It is known that many of the babies from these "forced" pregnancies are born prematurely, are often small, not strong and some have life-long disabilities. If, due to tubal damage, IVF is absolutely necessary, Foresight prepare both parents first, and then suggest natural cycle, drug free, treatment.

THE WAY FORWARD

Looking at nature as a whole, it seems that it is normal for reproduction to take place where conditions are optimal, and to fail where the environment is non-accommodating or hostile. At Foresight, we believe that, by working with nature, we can reverse a lot of the ill-health trends of the last few disastrous decades, especially in the field of reproduction.

INFERTILITY AND SUBFERTILITY

"78% of 'infertile' couples (compared with 20% with IVF alone) have been helped to have a healthy baby with the Foresight prgramme"

On the Foresight Programme we see low sperm counts increasing to normal quite regularly, and often hear of "polycystic" ovaries starting to ovulate again. This is achieved once nutrient levels are optimised, and toxins lowered following a hair mineral analysis and appropriate supplementation.

Blocked tubes we tackle with a four point plan: with homœopathy to cope with the infection; reflexology to increase the peristaltic action to clear the mucus and pus; the omission of cow's milk from the diet to combat the catarrhal aspect; and zinc and other nutrients as required according to the hair mineral analysis to increase general fertility.

In some cases, the sides of the tubes may have grown together, making repair impossible. In these cases, IVF will be necessary. Two count-ups of couples going for IVF after the Foresight Programme have shown success rates of 59% and 47% (as against the national average of 20%).

Foresight can introduce you to Nutritional Therapists who can help you with your diet, including detecting and coping with allergies and intestinal parasites if you need this.

We are also in touch with reflexologists who know how to help stimulate hormone levels. They can often help to unblock fallopian tubes, and re-activate sluggish ovaries. Not to mention helping the male partner by waking up the sperm beds to remind them what they are meant to be doing! This will increase production of mobile sperm in most cases.

Experienced osteopaths, naturopaths, reflexologists, homœopaths and acupuncturists can often stimulate hormonal systems by activating the pineal and the pituitary glands, thus achieving an ovulation.

Homœopaths can give the "whole person" (you!) a general boost, and can provide "nosodes" and other potentised remedies to combat infections and parasites.

Foresight Clinicians and Practitioners work privately, charges vary according to location. It is usual and acceptable to inquire about the charges when you ring to make an appointment.

THE FORESIGHT PROGRAMME

Foresight has worked since 1978 to put together a thoroughly researched preconception programme.

The work was based on research from all around the world, particularly from America, Canada and Australia. This has been augmented by our own experience, working closely with clients from all walks of life and ethnic groups, and each couple who has become close to us, and shared their life story with us, has added to the sum of knowledge. We are delighted to share this with you, to help you build your own unique and wonderful family.

A summary of the overall Foresight Programme follows, for more detailed information on each area see the relevant section in the booklet.

PART ONE — NUTRITION

It is essential that both prospective parents eat an excellent diet for at least four months before conception. Couples are advised to buy organic foods whenever possible. We advise filtering the drinking water to avoid toxic metals, agrochemicals and excess chlorine and oestrogens. Foresight registered nutritional therapists are available to help put together an eating programme to help you achieve an optimum diet. (See page 9).

PART TWO — HAIR ANALYSIS AND SUPPLEMENT PROGRAMMES

Arguably hair mineral analysis is the most important aspect of the whole programme. This can reveal both high levels of toxins, such as lead and cadmium, which can be disastrous to fetal development; and also low levels of essential elements. These deficiencies can also be harmful. Either problem can result in malformations or mental problems. Both can be corrected *in advance of pregnancy* using hair analysis and appropriate supplementation. (See page 14).

PART THREE — HEALTH & LIFESTYLE ADVICE

ALCOHOL, TOBACCO AND STREET DRUGS

Both partners need to be informed of the dangers of smoking, alcohol and street drugs to the health and development of the sperm and ova, and to the future fetus. Both partners are advised to abstain for at least four months prior to conception. (See page 22).

GENITO-URINARY AND OTHER INFECTIONS

It is advisable for both partners to be checked out for any genito–urinary infections.

In a recent survey of both partners in a London clinic, 69% were found to have at least one genito-urinary infection. In another survey 81% of the women were found to have one or more conditions. These can often be a symptomless infection that will only be activated by the hormonal stimulation of pregnancy.

Untreated, these conditions can lead to infertility, a series of miscarriages, or to premature and sickly babies. (See page 28).

FAMILY PLANNING

Where the woman has been using the contraceptive pill (or hormonal IUD) mineral levels will need to be tested and corrected. (The pill lowers zinc, manganese, vitamin A and the B-complex vitamins.)

Natural Family Planning by fertility awareness, with the use of barriers in the fertile phase, is suggested as the method of choice and should ideally be used for at least 4 months prior to conception. (See page 30).

ALLERGIES AND PARASITES

Allergy and intolerance to specific foods or inhalants can be responsible for a wide variety of illnesses inlcuding asthma, eczema, migraine, insomnia, depression, irritable bowel syndrome and coeliac disease. With dietary manipulation a lot of medication that is contraindicated in pregnancy may be avoided.

Parasitic infestations such as Giardia lamblia may also be present. Herbal or homœopathic treatment is recommended. Where parasites are eliminated the absorption of essential nutrients will be much improved. Where the history reveals a chronic problem likely to be incompatible with a healthy pregnancy, specialist help is recommended. (See page 33).

ELECTROMAGNETIC RADIATION

We are learning more all the time about the dangers of the various types of radiation and electromagnetic pollution. As this becomes increasingly intrusive, due to the proliferation of domestic gadgets, mobile phone masts, etc, we need to become more aware of the dangers and how to avoid them. Luckily, it is becoming easier to combat at home, as new aids are being developed, such as screening nets, metal-free mattresses and foil sandwich wallpaper. (See page 35).

OTHER HAZARDS

These constantly come to light, such as the toxic substances found in many household products and food processing and fluoride in the drinking water. Over 200 toxic substances have recently been discovered in the amniotic fluid of pregnant mothers: as more chemicals are introduced, we must become ever more watchful and aware. (See page 36).

PART ONE — NUTRITION

"Hormonal or vitamin imbalances which cause malaise or even pass unnoticed in postnatal life, may have a disastrous effect on the developing fetus. Interference with growth or metabolism of developing cells at an early stage is reflected ultimately in alterations at the stage of differentiation, with resulting malformations or impaired function of developing organs and tissues"   (Isobel Jennings, 1972).

Nutrition underpins every aspect of health. Research done by a number of eminent workers in the field of nutrition and fetal development has demonstrated the vital link. The work of Isobel Jennings, Weston Price, E.J. Underwood, Donald Oberleas, Donald Caldwell, Lucille Hurley, Bert Vallee, Carl Pfeiffer, Elizabeth Lodge-Rees, Richard Passwater, Elmer Cranton, Roger Williams, Arthur and Margaret Wynn, James Riordon and many others has drawn attention to the role played by lack of nutrients in reproductive disaster in experimental situations.

Almost all the commonly seen birth defects, (spina bifida and other neural tube defects, heart defects, diaphragmatic hernia, urogenital anomalies, cleft palate, club foot, missing digits and so on) can be reproduced or eliminated at will by manipulating the diet in animal studies. The removal of even one essential nutrient during the crucial first trimester of pregnancy can produce a characteristic defect that can be seen in different species, and in whole litters of young. In the same animals, the situation can be reversed in subsequent litters with replacement of the nutrient.

In this research, it was also demonstrated that problems such as sterility, spontaneous abortion, premature birth, and undersized young can be produced or eliminated at will by dietary intervention.

For too long all of this research has been reported only in the medical literature, while identical tragedies have continued to plague the human race.

Recently, the NACNE report has stressed the wisdom of eating more whole grains, vegetables and fruit, and criticised the high consumption of sugar in the UK. This is a step in the right direction – but too little – and very late.

THE OPTIMUM DIET

The optimum diet is to vary the foods by choosing each day from the 4 main food groups, while keeping as closely as possible to fresh whole foods.

CEREALS

100% Wholegrain flour, bread, pasta, cereals, muesli, porridge, crispbreads and brown rice. Use whole rye, barley, oats, millet, buckwheat, sesame, sunflower seeds and nuts. Be sure to find organic supplies, these will not contain toxic residues of fertilisers and pesticides and not be GM contaminated.

However, grains are difficult to digest. They need to have their complex starches such as phytates, broken down before being eaten, which will then allow for improved digestion and absorption of minerals such as calcium, zinc, iron and many others.

Phytates/phytic acid found in the bran of grains, binds to minerals and interferes with their absorption leading to a depletion of minerals in the body. Soaking grains or muesli overnight in an acid medium such as buttermilk or yoghurt, may substantially inactivate the phytates by morning, making the grain more digestible.

Most shop bought bread uses yeast as a raising agent, but this is not as good a degrader of phytates as sourdough.

DAIRY PRODUCTS

Whole milk, butter, cheese, yoghurt, fromage frais. If you suffer from allergies such as eczema or asthma you should consider cutting out cow's milk products, at least for a few weeks to see if there is a problem with them. Some people are more tolerant of goat and sheep products. There appear to be a growing number of lactose intolerant people who need to use dairy type products from a vegetable source, such as rice, oats, nuts or soya.

VEGETABLES, FRUITS AND JUICES

All fresh fruit and vegetables should preferably be eaten raw, or very lightly cooked, except for potatoes and pulses which need to be well cooked. If fruit is stewed, avoid aluminium saucepans, as they release a lot of toxic metal into the juice.

Choose vegetable and fruit juices that are free from sugar and colourings.

It is now easy to find organically grown produce; all supermarkets have a well stocked organic section and there are plenty of excellent farmer's markets and box schemes throughout the country. For those with space to grow fruit and vegetables, Lawrence Hills' little book, "Organic Gardening" is a classic. To grow, pick and eat ensures freshness as well as freedom from chemicals. It also saves money and food miles!

PROTEIN FOODS

All meats, poultry, game and fish, especially shellfish and roe. Eggs, dairy produce, pulses, seeds and nuts. Meat should be bought and eaten as fresh as possible. Keep to organic produce to avoid the risk of hormones, antibiotics, growth enhancers and GMOs.

Foods where the animal has been in its natural environment, such as venison, pheasant and most fish are good buys. However, until Government sources can assure us that the dangers of listeria and salmonella are past, soft cheeses and pates should be avoided in preconception and pregnancy, and hen's eggs should be well cooked.

> N.B. Unfortunately at this juncture in time we have to warn against organ meats such as liver and kidneys because of the possibility of accumulated toxins in them, and because of listeria. This also applies to liver and other pates. Due to the present dangers of both listeria and salmonella, protein foods should be well cooked, as this will destroy possible pathogens.

OTHER FOOD ISSUES

"Tampering with the food sources" as described by Dr Ferguson, can take many forms. Each may inhibit the use of some vital nutrient, of remove it from the body. Traditional hazards include environmental lead and cadmium, artificial fertilisers, antibiotics, some food additives (sweeteners, colourings, flavourings etc), organophosphate pesticides, fluoride in water and many others. Now add to this depressing list genetic modification.

Filtering both drinking and cooking water, in order to remove lead, and excess copper, pesticides, oestrogens and chlorine, is necessary.

The work of the late Dr. Feingold of California demonstrated the effect on small children of many artificial colourings and other additives used to render more acceptable the stale denatured food of the tin, jar and packet. Dr. Feingold found that many additives were at least a contributory cause of hyperactivity and learning difficulties.

More detailed research into the effects of tartrazine showed it to lower levels of zinc in the body by increasing urinary excretion (Ward 1992). Further research may reveal this to be common to other additives which share the clinical effects. As these additives have been shown to affect brain function and zinc status in a school age child, we can assume they will affect the unborn. (Most problem children improve enormously in health and behaviour once additives are removed from the diet and supplements of zinc and manganese are given.) We cannot advise too strongly that effort is made to avoid additives in the preconceptual period and during pregnancy and breast feeding. See our booklet "FIND OUT" for further information.

Allergic illness, and conditions such as Candida albicans, can impair absorption. Infection can stress the immune system, squandering nutrients such as zinc, and Vitamins A and C. Stress also depletes reserves of nutrients, as does smoking, alcohol and oral contraception.

THE IMPORTANCE OF TRACE ELEMENTS

The important role of trace elements in health and reproduction is becoming clearer each decade as research in this area becomes more sophisticated. It is likely that many more factors associated with nutrient metabolism have yet to be discovered. Basing the diet as much as possible on whole fresh foods, grown organically on healthy soil, is a sensible way to help to optimise nutritional status. This strategy will help us to cover the probable many factors about which there is as yet no documentation.

However, we do not all have space to grow things, and much manufactured food will have been stored for some time before reaching the consumer. Custom dictates that foods such as meat are cooked and milk is pasteurised, and much commercial food will be raised on poor soil lacking in trace minerals, so many nutrients may still be in less than optimum supply, even in apparently healthy food.

For this reason in 1979 Foresight nutritional advisors, headed by Prof. John Dickerson, then professor of Human Nutrition at Surrey University, formulated some well balanced vitamin and mineral supplements, to be used in conjunction with the diet as described.

With the help of Dr. Robert Woodward, Foresight formulated additional supplements in capsule form, consisting of the index nutrient, supported by the nutrients involved in its metabolism, packed in organic vegetable powder. These we recommend where indicated by the hair analysis.

We believe this has made a major contribution to the success of the Foresight Programme in protecting against all forms of reproductive hazard, also contributing to the health and to subsequent successful breast-feeding, and thus to the complete emotional fulfilment of our mothers.

Nutrition generally is a huge subject and cannot be covered adequately in a small book. We recommend our other publications which includes our Wholefood Diet Leaflet and Foresight Wholefood Cookbook.

PART TWO —
HAIR ANALYSIS
& SUPPLEMENT
PROGRAMMES

Foresight provides laboratory facilities for hair analyses to establish the presence of excess heavy (toxic) metals or the shortage of minerals and essential trace elements.

Where both minerals and essential trace elements are shown to be below the optimum for healthy fetal development we give a programme of supplementation for a stated period, then retest. Similarly, where the toxic metals are above the threshold level for safety for fetal development, we give a cleansing programme of Vitamin C, Garlic and Vitamins B1 and B12 until they are within the safe limits.

The supplement / cleansing programme is adjusted and repeated until levels compatible with a healthy pregnancy are achieved. This usually takes about 4 - 8 months.

Following the full programme, the pregnancy can be started with normal, strong sperm and egg, the embryo can implant in a healthy uterus and can develop in optimum conditions. There will be no danger from nutritional deficiency, or damage from heavy metals or other toxins or viral and / or bacterial disease. Foresight has found that under these conditions it is possible to have uncomplicated pregnancies resulting in strong, healthy and perfectly formed babies.

HAIR ANALYSIS

When you visit a Foresight Practitioner they will take a hair sample to send in for analysis. Alternatively you can contact Foresight directly and they will give you instructions for taking your own hair sample to send in with the appropriate fee. The hair will be analysed at the Foresight laboratory, and an interpretation of the analysis will be sent as a programme of the supplements you need, along with a letter explaining how to proceed.

The supplements will aim to reduce any toxic metals that are revealed, and will supplement any minerals and trace elements that are seen to be deficient.

Hair analysis gives a good, rough guide to mineral status. At Foresight we have 29 years of successful experience using the technique (1978-2007). The Foresight laboratory uses a modern ICP-MS instrument. They currently test hair, tap water, shampoos, herbal remedies, supplements, etc. The full range of tests can be very helpful under special circumstances, and the findings are also useful from the point of view of research. We prefer hair to any other sample. The body fluids (blood, saliva, urine and sweat) being in a constant state of flux, vary around the day. The hair, however, gives approximately an eight week history of the minerals absorbed. If the hair samples are correctly taken, any variations between repeat samples are very small, and unlikely to affect levels of supplementation.

Minerals below the Recommended Values need to be supplemented to optimum levels (i.e. at or above the guidelines shown). High levels of toxic metals above the Threshold Values need to be reduced.

HEAVY METAL POLLUTION

Lead and cadmium pollution have been linked in a number of studies to infertility, miscarriage, prematurity, low birth weight, perinatal death and malformation; also to stunted growth and to learning and co-ordination difficulties in older children. From the outset Foresight has analysed hair samples prior to pregnancy. We like to see lead below 1.4ppm, cadmium below 0.14ppm, aluminium below 2ppm and mercury below 0.14ppm.

In trying to lower the body burden of heavy metal, or an over-high level of copper, it is important to trace the sources of contamination, and lower or correct these if possible, as well as taking steps to lower the level in the body.

Useful nutrients for cleansing the body of heavy metals are Vitamin C, Milk Thistle and Garlic, Vitamins B_1, B_3 and B_{12} (formulated as "Vitamin C and Garlic")and the essential minerals calcium, magnesium, iron, zinc, manganese and selenium. Where indicated, we use Nicotinamide as an additional liver cleanser.

LEAD

Lead comes from flaking paint and dust from this, and from water, due to lead piping or lead-glazed earthenware mains, and occasionally from occupational hazards such as powdered ink, artist's paint, leaded ties as in stained glass windows. Builders especially can be at risk from scraping down old paint, and from cement and roofing felt.

Tap water can be tested by the Foresight laboratory to find out if the levels of lead, mercury, copper, cadmium and aluminium are within the EU limits (although we'd suggest lower limits). We recommend you filter drinking and cooking water.

Old paint may contain lead: when stripping down, wear protective clothing including covering face and hair, and rubber gloves, and wet down the working area frequently.

MERCURY

The most common mercury contamination we find is from dental amalgam. Amalgam fillings continuously leach small amounts of mercury that makes its way into the blood stream. However, unless you have a lot of mercury fillings, or your hair mineral analysis shows high levels of mercury toxicity in your system, it is probably best to leave the fillings in situ because the process of removing them will release even higher levels of mercury into your system for a period of time.

Dental patients void mercury in the urine for up to eight days after repairs with mercury amalgams. Discuss with your dentist alternative materials for future dental repairs which also need to be free from fluoride. Dentists/dental nurses are also at risk and it will also help them if patients insist on mercury-free fillings!

Mercury is also found in tuna fish and swordfish and in water that is contaminated by agriculture (seed wheat is dusted with mercury), also from some weedkillers.

Avoid eating tuna or swordfish, and handling seed-wheat and weedkillers.

Cadmium

Cadmium comes from cigarette smoke, self-inflicted or passive smoking, and in some areas from drinking water contaminated by industrial practices or rubbish disposal.

Burning old rubber tyres is another source. Beware motor race tracks! Avoid smoking and, where possible, smoky atmospheres.

Aluminium

Aluminium comes from cookware, pressure cookers, kettles and teapots. Tannin will complex with aluminium, and leach it into the tea. Foil saucers and foil wraps contaminate on contact. Some milk substitutes, salt and baking powder contain silico-aluminate. Some salt is in aluminium-lined containers. Many deodorants contain aluminium. There are several excellent natural, organic alternatives which are free from aluminium.

Some antacids have 500mg of aluminium per tablet, other antacids are aluminium-free (e.g. herbal based ones). Water Authorities often use aluminium gel during the purification process, which may impart the metal to the water.

Change aluminium cookware, avoid using foil. Check labels for additives in food and medications. Filter drinking water.

Over-high Copper

Copper is an essential trace element. However, too heavy contamination from copper piping, combined with the use of the copper IUD, the Pill, and/or long-term use of hormones such as Clomid, etc. (which cause the body to retain copper) can cause levels to rise to far above the normal range.

Where the water is soft and acid, copper may be leached from the pipes. Copper may be released from new pipes for several years. Copper pipes joined to old lead connecting pipes, or two copper pipes joined by lead-containing solder, may corrode and release both metals into the water. Water heaters may release copper from the small gauge piping, so kettles should not be filled from these.

Other sources are copper kettles and pans, hair dyes, copper-containing algicides in swimming pools and possibly brass jewellery.

Foresight advises Natural Family Planning as the preferred choice for birth control, with barriers during the fertile phase; the use of water filters for all drinking and cooking water; and alternative types of algicide in pools. Choose a different, non-copper-containing hair colouring if you dye your hair regularly.

OVER-HIGH SELENIUM

Selenium is an essential trace element. However, over-high levels can be toxic and can result from using anti-dandruff selenium shampoos too frequently, or in the bath. The maker's instructions should be adhered to.

We would advise against their use entirely during preconception and pregnancy.

MINERAL DEFICIENCIES AND SUPPLEMENTATION

Research from America and Australia has highlighted the dangers of mineral deficiencies in pregnancy. Work with experimental animals has shown that deficiencies can cause a wide variety of malformations and lack of mental acuity, and also an increase in premature birth and perinatal mortality.

COPPER BALANCE

Copper rises gently in the mother's blood throughout the pregnancy. The work of Professor Bert Vallee of Harvard University Medical School, with zinc/copper ratios in rats showed that during the third trimester of pregnancy, zinc was packed into the placental tissue, so the ratio of copper to zinc rose in the blood. Vallee found that when the ratio of copper to zinc rose to a certain level, the phenomena of birth was stimulated. Subsequently, he observed that, as the rats ate the placenta after birth, the zinc/copper ratio was restored to normal in both mother and young by 96 hours after birth. Too high a level of copper/too low a level of zinc too soon in pregnancy, runs the risk of stimulating this response too early, resulting in miscarriage or premature birth. Zinc and copper levels need to be monitored and adjusted throughout the pregnancy.

ZINC

After the birth, there is a case to be made for supplementing ALL new mothers with zinc to compensate for not consuming the placenta. Professor Bryce-Smith of Reading University, found normal placentas contain 360-600mg of zinc. We suggest 60mg a day for at least 10 days after birth. This helps the breastmilk to arrive and has a calming effect on mother and baby. It also helps to heal any abrasions and combat possible infection.

It is important that zinc levels are optimised preconceptually, throughout the pregnancy, during breast-feeding and subsequently in the child, as a zinc-deficient child is at risk to eczema, asthma, diarrhoea and later learning difficulties – hyperactivity, dyslexia, etc. The immune system is compromised (since it is zinc dependant), and it is likely that this is a contributory factor in certain cases of autism. Many "problem children" suffer from what could be called "sub-clinical autism", and which responds favourably to the normalisation of mineral status.

The seeds of disaffection, difficult behaviour, later truancy, delinquency and criminality can be sown in these very early days. So much family agony and public horror and expense could be pre-empted, if the work of these early researchers was taken on board and the baby's brain function and total well-being was given the consideration it deserves.

Work done in USA by Weston Price, Roger Williams, Bert Vallee, Carl Pfeiffer, Unabelle Blackwood, Elizabeth Lodge-Rees, Donald Caldwell & Donald Oberleas, Lucille Hurley, Richard Passwater, Elmer Cranton; that done in Australia by E.J. Underwood; and in this country by Professor D. Bryce-Smith, Dr Niel Ward and Isobel Jennings, has revealed a wide range of ills suffered as a result of mineral difficiencies in both human and experimental situations. Sterility, abortion, stillbirth, infant deaths, many types of malformation, hyperactivity and lack of mental acuity have all been demonstrated to be attributable to mineral deficiencies.

Hyperemesis, post-partum depression, lack of mother-baby bonding and lactation failure, also restlessness (screaming!) and failure of the baby to thrive, have all been linked to deficiencies of zinc, manganese, magnesium, Vitamin B6 and essential fatty acids.

ZINC AND FERTILITY

Low levels of zinc have been found to be responsible for implantation failure, and it is probable that the zinc loss sustained during the first pregnancy is sometimes a cause of subsequent subfertility. Down the years, Foresight has found that unexplained subfertility almost always responds to supplementation with zinc and other needed trace elements.

Male infertility also often responds to mineral supplementation by restoring levels found to be low by hair mineral analyses. (Also correcting high levels of toxic metals, and eliminating smoking, alcohol, genito-urinary infections and the use of mobile phones).

OTHER CONSIDERATIONS

Where a number of minerals and essential trace elements are found to be low, or there is a very ragged pattern, this may indicate a condition such as coeliac disease, cow's milk allergy, intestinal parasites such as Giardia, Candida or threadworms. This should be investigated and treated appropriately with homœopathic or herbal preparations. Inadequate diet may be part of the story, and a previous history of anorexia/bulimia may manifest in this way. Your Foresight Practitioner can work at this with you, to get things back to normal.

A low level of sodium and/or potassium is said to indicate stress or poor adrenal function. Dietary adjustment to eliminate allergens is helpful. Magnesium-pantothenate supplementation can help to normalise adrenal function.

A high level of sodium and potassium has been linked to kidney/urinary tract infections. It may also be present when kidneys and liver are irritated by high quantities of heavy metals passing through.

After the pill, the copper IUD, ovulation-stimulating drugs (Clomid, etc), previous childbirth, or problems with tap water, copper may be over-high. Being biochemically antagonistic, zinc, and possibly also magnesium and manganese may be too low, as copper will push them out of the body. It is vital to adjust this before embarking on the next pregnancy, to avoid the risk of miscarriage or premature birth.

CAUSES OF LOW MINERAL LEVELS

Possible reasons for low levels of minerals are manifold:

- Zinc and copper are biochemical antagonists. Copper from water pipes is a common cause of low zinc.
- Zinc may be low after use of the pill, other exogenous hormones (which cause the body to retain copper), or the copper coil.
- Zinc, manganese and selenium become reduced as a result of lead and/or copper contamination from whatever source.
- All minerals are reduced in foodstuffs as a result of modern agricultural practices which strip the soil of minerals.
- Smoking and/or alcohol stress liver function, and this squanders zinc and B complex vitamins.
- Zinc is used by the immune system. This means it will be lower after stress, injury, surgery or infectious illness, including hidden genito-urinary infections.
- Food allergies and coeliac condition can inhibit the uptake of nutrients. Thus long-standing illness of this type can result in multiple deficiencies.
- All minerals will be reduced by intestinal parasites.
- Previous anorexia, "slimming" by skipping meals etc, can reduce minerals.
- Chromium and cobalt tend to be low where the diet contains much sugar and/or alcohol, and cobalt may be low in vegetarians who may lack vitamin B12.
- Manganese absorption may be reduced by organophosphate pesticides (which prevent it crossing the gut/blood barrier); it is also thought to be lowered by the pill. Manganese is essential to make thyroxine. Thyroid function is inhibited by fluoride, so fluoride in toothpaste might cause over-use of manganese.
- Magnesium levels are also thought to be reduced by the pill, and by fluoride from water and fluoridated toothpaste.
- Refined (white) flour and sugar are very low in all minerals and B vitamins. They therefore tend to steal them from the body's reserves, as carbohydrate metabolism uses up more minerals than these de-natured foods are able to provide. The calories provided by these foods are commonly referred to as "empty calories". Constant use of empty calories will gradually erode the body's mineral reserves.

PROBLEM SOLVING

Where couples have a history of infertility or problems with previous pregnancies, Foresight has found there are almost invariably mineral imbalances which have to be reversed before a successful pregnancy will be achieved. This is an integral part of the full Foresight Programme and contributes largely to our successful record.

Vitamin and mineral regimes have been used since 1979 by Foresight with consistently excellent results, as is shown by our recent research study.

More specific information can be found in Foresight literature and on the website, including the manifestations of ill-health directly attributable to mineral deficiencies in adults and children.

PART THREE — HEALTH & LIFESTYLE ADVICE

ALCOHOL, TOBACCO AND STREET DRUGS

ALCOHOL

Alcohol can have a detrimental effect on fertility, pregnancy and health. Foresight strongly urges BOTH parents to avoid alcohol before and during pregnancy for your health and for that of your child to be.

Effects on Fertility

'Women warned to avoid alcohol when trying to conceive'

This headline followed the release of research that found that women drinking 5 units or less a week were twice as likely to conceive within six months than women drinking 10 units or more. (British Medical Journal, 1998). **Then, the same year, an article in "Fertility and Sterility" found that alcohol AT ANY LEVEL significantly reduced fertility by up to 50%.**

Problems Caused by Alcohol During Pregnancy

- Growth abnormalities
- Cranio-facial abnormalities
- Musculoskeletal abnormalities
- Cardiac abnormalities
- Nervous system abnormalities
- Neurodevelopmental delay or mental deficiency
- Short stature which may be permanent

Learning and behavioural deficits are widely variable, including: Problems with co-operation, sustained attention, comprehension, retention of information, self-control, relationships, word recall, organisational skills.

The Solution

Avoidance of alcohol by both partners for at least 4 months prior to pregnancy to ensure undamaged sperm and ova, and, for the woman, throughout pregnancy and breastfeeding.

Further Information

Pregnant women have been advised to avoid alcohol in traditional societies and in our culture since biblical times, however it wasn't until 1973 that fetal alcohol syndrome (FAS) was to be defined by a group of medical researchers in USA, and interest was re-awakened.

Fetal alcohol syndrome has now been more clearly defined by international research and the full abnormalities are accepted to be: underweight and under length at birth; slow growth and failure to thrive after birth even with special postnatal care; unusually small head with defective development of mid-facial tissues; joint and limb abnormalities; possible mental retardation, dyslexia, and/or "behavioural problems" such as hyperactivity and extreme nervousness.

Alcohol crosses the placental barrier freely and travels through the baby's bloodstream in the same concentration as that present in the mother's.

In the National Council of Women's Report, 1976, which provided this information, Dr. David Woollams of Cambridge, and Dr. Richard Bast of the NIAAA of USA both stated that the only safe limit for pregnancy was no alcohol at all.

Since then, Dr. Anne Streissguth of Washington has described the condition Fetal Alcohol Effect (FAE). This term is given to babies less impaired than those with FAS, but whose intelligence, behaviour and growth have been significantly retarded by parental alcohol consumption. Seven year olds whose mothers had one drink daily during pregnancy were found to have a 7 point IQ deficit. Dr. Streissguth followed affected babies through to adulthood, and found that problems were compounded rather than resolved as they grew older.

A number of reports have demonstrated that alcohol can be particularly harmful to men and women before conception (damage to sperm and ova), and to women and unborn children during the first 4-5 months of pregnancy.

In 1983. Dr. Matthew Kaufman of Cambridge drew attention to the dangers of "a single episode of heavy drinking by the mother at about the time of conception". Alcohol given to female mice immediately after mating caused severe damage to the chromosomes of one/fifth to one/sixth of the eggs. This could result in spontaneous abortion, or death shortly after birth. Much abnormality in human young can be traced back to chromosomal abnormalities.

For total safety and optimum development in the child, Foresight advocates a complete embargo on alcohol for both parents in the four months leading up to the intended conception, and for the mother throughout pregnancy and breast-feeding. The benefits to the child will be immeasurable. The benefits to the nation will be vast. It is likely at the moment (2007) that more than half the population will be functioning at much below their true potential, which is so unnecessary. Most of it is simply due to lack of information getting to those who need it most at the right time.

For people who find it really hard to give up alcohol, the following may be useful:

- Alcohol interferes with biochemical pathways that assist the assimilation of important fats. These fats are used for brain function and disruption can result in muddled thinking, loss of competence and depression. It is helpful to take fish oils, which are rich in Omega 3 and essential fatty acids, to compensate.
- Alcohol also disturbs the body's ability to handle sugars. This can result in very violent mood swings and alienating behaviour. Supplementing with B complex Vitamins and zinc, manganese and chromium will help get things back to normal.
- Alcohol puts a huge demand on the liver. Much alcohol related illness is due to exhausted liver function. Supplementing with Vitamin C, B_{12}, B_1 and B_3, also garlic and milk thistle, will help to cleanse the liver.

I often see questionnaires where people are drinking what would be considered "moderately" (within Government guidelines!) 14-21 units a week, but who nevertheless tick the box for depression, or say they are taking anti depressants. Not everybody realises that drinking alcohol is usually followed by a period of depression, and that giving it up solves a lot of problems for a lot of people! (Not least the relatives!)

SMOKING

In 1980 the report of the USA Surgeon-General *"The Health Consequences of Smoking for Women"* demonstrated that smoking is a major cause of abnormalities in pregnancies, and avoidable illness and deformity in children.

In 1957 Simpson reported that babies born to smokers were on average 200gms lighter. 45 studies have confirmed that smoking is a major cause of low birth weight. The more a woman smokes, the greater is the reduction in birthweight. Smokers have nearly twice the risk of spontaneous abortion, and the risks of premature birth rise with the number of cigarettes smoked from 6% for non-smokers, through 11% for smokers who use 10 cigarettes a day, to 33% (one baby in 3) where mothers smoke 30 cigarettes a day.

The neo-natal death rate also rises directly with the number of cigarettes smoked. Smokers' placentas tend to be thinner and most of these unnecessary deaths are due to placental haemorrhages causing premature delivery.

Studies have found that smokers are also more likely to give birth to babies with all types of congenital abnormalities, especially cleft lip and palate, and central nervous system abnormalities. This risk is more than doubled in heavy smokers. Long term studies have shown reduced growth, learning difficulties, neurological abnormalities and abnormal EEGs, which may mean epilepsy and/or hyperactivity. Passive smoking by the baby after birth increases the risk of cot death, hyperactivity and asthma.

Children of heavily smoking fathers are more than twice as likely to have malformations. In men, smoking levels affect spermatogenesis (sperm development), sperm morphology (abnormality) and sperm mobility. Studies have shown that numbers of damaged sperm, and also the number of children born with a malformation, rise directly in line with the number of cigarettes smoked per day.

The number of children later suffering/dying from cancer or leukaemia also rises commensurably with the number of cigarettes smoked per day by the father prior to their conception.

In research sponsored by the Teratology Committee of the German Research Council it was found that not only serious congenital malformations but perinatal mortality was significantly higher among the babies of smoking fathers, after correcting for the effects on pregnancy outcome of mothers' smoking and the possible effects of eleven other factors. When even 10 cigarettes a day were smoked, the chances of malformation were increased by over 2.5 times.

Fathers' daily cigarette consumption	Malformed babies per 1,000
Zero	8.22
1 – 10	13.8
over 10	21.2

Paternal cigarette consumption and occurrence of severe congenital malformations.
Based on 5,183 births, Germany 1974

Even after birth, additional health problems burden smokers' children. A Report by the Royal College of Physicians in 1992 said that children whose parents or carers smoke may inhale the equivalent of 60-150 cigarettes a year and are more likely to have glue ear and twice as likely to have breathing difficulties, asthma and infections.

STREET DRUGS

Street drugs can have a detrimental effect on fertility, pregnancy and health. Foresight strongly urges BOTH parents to avoid any kind of street drugs, both for your health and for that of your offspring.

CANNABIS / MARIJUANA

> *"Marijuana's impairing cellular effects on DNA can result in incomplete genetic information being transmitted to the offspring"*.   Dr Gabriel Nahas

Cannabis is four times more dangerous to your health than cigarette smoking. It dumps three times more tar in the lungs and five times more carbon monoxide.

The key psychoactive substance in cannabis is tetrahydrocannabinol (THC) – this component has the same steroid structure found in the sex hormones and in certain hormones of the adrenal glands. THC accumulates in the ovaries and testes.

In women cannabis can upset the menstrual cycle. In men it lowers blood testosterone, lowers sperm count, causes greater than usual impotency and diminished libido. Sperm motility is also affected and there is an increase in number of abnormal sperm.

Cannabis effects the synthesis of DNA – whether used by the man or woman. In animals, studies have demonstrated the link with increased fetal deaths and malformations.

COCAINE & CRACK

In mice cocaine is proven to be teratogenic i.e. it causes malformations to the fetus even at non-toxic levels to the mother. In humans there is a decrease in the weight of the fetus, a higher malformation rate and increased still birth rate.

Crack is a cocaine derivative which is purer than cocaine. It also causes malformations, and the *withdrawal symptoms in the newborn are severe.*

HEROIN

Heroin and other opiate narcotics such as opium, morphine and codeine are all extremely addictive.

They cause decreased fertility and atrophy of the male sex organs, as well as decreased testosterone.

Heroin addicts experience:
- 3 times more stillbirths
- 4 times more premature births
- 6 times more growth problems in the fetus

Also babies are born addicted to the drug and have to endure withdrawal.

GENITO-URINARY AND OTHER INFECTIONS

The radical changes in sexual behaviour over the last few decades have resulted in a dramatic rise in the prevalence of sexually transmitted infections. Whilst the classical venereal diseases such as syphilis and gonorrhoea are in decline due to early detection and treatment, their place has been taken by groups of other infections. In recent years, the Chlamydia pathogen, has been found to manifest as cervicitis, endometritis, acute salpingitis and pelvic inflammatory disease.

It has also been found directly responsible for ectopic pregnancy, prematurity, perinatal mortality and spontaneous abortion. In addition, Chlamydia trachomatis infection is directly implicated as one of the most common causes of infertility.

In infants, Chlamydial infection is associated with a myriad of clinical conditions including: Pneumonitis, Conjunctivitis, Otitis media, Gastro-enteritis, Viral disease and other conditions. It may be a good idea to ask for a urine test for infants known to be at risk.

In men, Chlamydial infection is recognised as the leading cause of epididymitis and urethritis, as well as contributing to male infertility or subfertility.

The spread of other infections which are also frequently sexually transmitted such as viruses and mycoplasmas has also grown to near epidemic proportions. Maternal mycoplasma infections have been associated with a high incidence of spontaneous abortions and prematurity as well as neonatal morbidity and mortality. All types of genito-urinary infection are shown to contribute to infertility, miscarriage and premature birth. *Due to the prevalence of these diseases in the general population, Foresight advocates routinely testing every couple as part of the preconception care work-up.*

From 109 patients who attended one Foresight Clinician, 76 had an infection (69%), or roughly 2 out of 3. Each of the conditions listed below were found in at least one patient:

Chlamydia	Heam.strep	Haem.influenza
Ureaplasma	Strep Millerii	Klebsiella
Mycoplasma	Staph.aureas	E.Coli
Anaerobic bacteria	Gardnerella	Candida
B.Strep	Enterococcus	

We suggest routinely screening for all of the above, where possible, before the start of a pregnancy.

Cytomegalovirus, Toxoplasmosis and Rubella immunity should also be included in the screenings, where this can be arranged. Although these illnesses are comparatively rare, they can result in blindness, deafness, epilepsy and retardation in the baby, so caution is justified. With the two former, a positive finding of antibodies does not necessarily mean the disease is active; a further test for IgM levels will elucidate this. If the disease is active however, pregnancy should be postponed and specialist help sought.

You can obtain screening through your local Genito-Urinary Medicine Clinic, (G.U.M. Clinic) at your local hospital. You do not need a doctor's referral. Ring for an appointment. You can show them the above paragraphs.

For an active genito-urinary infection there are two possible courses of action:

Either, to use an antibiotic which can be given by the G.U.M. Clinic or by your own G.P. Antibiotic use should always be followed by supplementation of vitamin B-complex, probiotics such as Acidophilus, and, for those who are not milk-allergic, the eating of live yoghurt to restore the intestinal flora and prevent the spread of Candida albicans.

Alternatively, we have found that many infections can be combated successfully with appropriate homœopathic remedies. Foresight can recommend a homœopathic practitioner. This method is preferable because it causes less damage to the intestinal flora and the immune system in general.

It is important that both partners follow a course of treatment, even if one of them appears to be symptom free due to the risks of cross infection. After either course of action, it is essential to retest at the G.U.M. Clinic to be sure the treatment has been effective.

FAMILY PLANNING

Natural Family Planning (NFP) provides an efficient means of fertility control which is non-invasive and therefore free from side-effects and health hazards. In the past, the main objection to this approach has been its reputed unreliability. The reasons for the high failure rates with the old "Calendar Rhythm Method" were irregular cycles and misinformation. This method must not be confused with the modern technique of NFP, which, on WHO statistics, has a biological failure rate of virtually zero!

It is now known that the egg, once it is shed from the ovary, is fertilisable for only 8 - 24 hours, but that sperm can live in the vagina for up to 6 days, given certain circumstances. The luteal phase (the time between ovulation and menstruation) can be as short as 10 days or as long as 16 days.

If a woman takes her temperature before rising for a few mornings each month, preferably with a special fertility thermometer, she will find her temperature at a lower level until she has ovulated. After ovulation her temperature will rise and stay at a higher level for the next two weeks. If she has conceived, her temperature will stay up providing proof of the pregnancy. If she has not conceived, it will fall with the onset of the period, and a new fertility cycle will start, repeating this biphasic temperature pattern.

There is a further sign, which is obvious to a woman, indicating that the egg is ripening in her ovary. As the egg-sac (follicle) starts ripening, a hormone called estrogen is produced which stimulates glands in the neck of the womb (cervix) to produce a clear and slippery mucus. This mucus is alkaline and neutralises the acidity of the vagina, enabling sperm to survive in it. It is rich in nutrients which attract and feed the sperm, prolonging their life. Its thin, watery nature provides a swimming lane through which the sperm can migrate into the cervix at incredible speed, and upwards towards the ripening egg. The mucus increases in flow for the 6 days that the follicle takes to ripen. It produces the sensation of lubrication of the vagina that women notice mid-cycle. Once in the mucus, the sperm can live for up to 6 days. Once the egg is released the production of mucus dries up and the womb cavity becomes ready to receive the baby.

When the mucus observation is combined with minimal use of the temperature method, the cycle can be accurately observed and understood. If a woman's cycle is regular, the ovulation pattern will also be regular. To control fertility, unprotected intercourse should be avoided on the day of ovulation and for 6 days prior to this date. When pregnancy is desired, intercourse during this period will allow conception to take place.

PROBLEMS FROM THE BIRTH CONTROL PILL

About 40% of women who take birth-control pills will have side effects of one kind or another during its use. Some of these side effects are: light bleeding between menstrual periods, skipped periods, nausea, weight change, bloating, increase in vaginal infections. A spotty darkening of the skin on the face may appear and may be permanent.

The most serious side effect associated with the birth-control pill is a greater chance of blood clots, stroke and heart attack. These problems occur in only a small number of women who take the pill. Other serious side effects are worsening of migraine headaches, gall bladder disease, depression or increased blood pressure. Potential long-term consequences to the child passed on from the mother having been on the pill prior to pregnancy are unknown.

Young women who take oral contraceptive pills before they become pregnant with their first child run a significantly higher risk of developing pre-menopausal breast cancer, according to new international research from Altoona Hospital in Pennsylvania.

COMING OFF THE PILL

Foresight advises all women to seek out an instructor of Natural Family Planning, so they can avoid the use of the contraceptive pill. It can cause the accumulation of copper in the woman's body, and use of the pill is being increasingly linked to breast cancer and other women's cancers.

In some cases it has caused migraine and feelings of being "over-stretched" throughout the month. With many women it has caused the onset of symptoms, thought to be due to allergy, or psychological factors. Luckily most of these misfortunes will reverse in a few months if the pill is dropped and the woman's nutrient levels are optimised.

We recommend that women come off the birth control pill for at least four months before trying to conceive and use natural birth control methods or barrier methods until conception. This will allow your body time to recover from having the artificial hormones flooding it and also give you time to improve your nutritional status.

FOR FURTHER INFORMATION:
- "Understanding Fertility" by Colleen Norman
  www.fertilityet.org.uk
- For help and advice ask your Foresight Branch Secretary for your Local NFP Teacher:

ALLERGIES AND PARASITES

It has been demonstrated that a wide variety of illnesses can be caused, wholly or in part, by allergic reactions.

These may range from trivial aches and pains, to many disabling physical conditions and mental disorders. Often these conditions can be alleviated by the removal of certain foods from the diet, or substances from the environment.

Dr. Vera Walker, then President of the British Association of Allergists, presented a paper in 1975 which showed the allergy prone family were particularly subject to dyslexia, hyperactivity, epilepsy and mental breakdown, as well as to commonly recognised allergic disorders such as hay fever, irritable bowel syndrome, asthma, eczema, migraine and insomnia.

Allergy is a complex subject. We have become increasingly aware of the interlinking between allergy and factors such as nutritional deficiencies, smoking, traffic effluent, pesticides, various food additives, intestinal parasites, hormonal disturbances from the contraceptive pill, gas, industrial pollutants, and geopathic stress. Infection, antibiotics and intestinal candida may also exacerbate conditions, and lack of zinc is known to undermine the immune system. Lessening the input from as many of these additional hazards as possible may help to lessen the severity of the allergic reaction.

THE LINK BETWEEN ALLERGY AND NUTRITION

Dr. Frank Pottenger of California did a most interesting study with cats. Cats in one run were fed cooked meat and pasteurised milk. They gave birth to kittens with narrow faces, underdeveloped jaws, running noses and poor fur; disadvantages that could be equated to allergic illness in humans. The cats in the second run were fed raw meat and whole milk. These cats gave birth to normal healthy kittens. This experiment would suggest that inadequate food prior to birth makes the offspring liable to facial malformations and allergic illness.

Dr. Lodge-Rees, a paediatrician from California, who worked with children with mental disorders and allergy, found many of her small allergic or retarded patients to have the narrow jaw and high raised palate described by Dr. Weston Price in "Nutrition and Physical Degeneration". This is a typical malformation resulting from poor diet before and after birth.

Subsequently, Dr. Lodge-Rees analysed the hair of many small patients and found those with the malformed face and allergic syndromes to be short of many minerals, and sometimes to have high levels of toxic metals.

EFFECTS ON THE FETUS

Many working in the field of allergy have found that the baby will be less liable to an allergic response if the mother is not eating substances to which she herself reacts during pregnancy and breast-feeding. Evidence is now accumulating to support this view. (In addition, avoidance of exposure to allergenic foods and environmental contaminants during the first year of life appears to reduce the likelihood of the baby developing allergic disease.)

It would seem wise to detect and eliminate allergens prior to conception, as (a) the substance will undermine the mother's general health, and this could adversely affect the course of the pregnancy, (b) allergy has often been found to increase pregnancy nausea and vomiting, and (c) the resolving of conditions such as eczema, asthma, migraine, epilepsy, insomnia, depression and so on, may mean a great many medical drugs can be discontinued or their use minimised. Many of these drugs may be contra-indicated in pregnancy, so this alternative form of control is to be welcomed.

ADDITIVES

It is quite possible to find someone reacts to a certain manufactured food, and then to discover that it is the additive(s) it contains that are to blame.

Foresight can supply the booklet "FIND OUT" that lists all the additives in current use, and the reactions that they can produce. This, and the companion booklet "WATCH IT", which lists toxic substances in toiletries and other household products are essential shopping aids!

SPECIALIST HELP

If, therefore, symptoms of chronic illness or malaise persist after discontinuing the contraceptive pill, smoking, hazardous food additives, filtering the water and reversing nutritional deficiencies, it is as well to seek specialist help in the field of allergy. A number of Foresight Clinicians work in this field.

Often, however, eliminating the most obvious foods, sometimes in "food families" can bring relief. It is worth starting with cow's milk and/or gluten.

Not all IBS (Irritable Bowel Syndrome) however, is caused by cow's milk allergy or coeliac condition. Some cases are due to intestinal parasites such as Giardia lamblia or Blastocitis hominis or some amoebic types of dysentery. Parasites can also be responsible for a wide range of seemingly auto-immune illnesses. This needs specialist help. We suggest contacting a nutritional therapist to arrange a stool sample to be sent for analysis.

Where parasites are eliminated the absorption of essential nutrients will be much improved, as will digestion and gut function.

ELECTROMAGNETIC RADIATION

The dangers of radiation from electric blankets, microwave ovens, sun-beds, VDUs, CB radios, luminous clocks, mobile phones and their masts and DECT phones are recognised. The effects on reproduction need to be more widely studied.

Some houses are built over "ley lines" and other sources of "rogue electricity" which emanate from cracks in granite substrata, or from under-ground rivers. These rivers often course through rock, and the water travelling along the edge of the rock-face can send up a strong electrical charge.

Since working together with Alfred and Roy Riggs, Foresight has become more aware of these issues. We refer people who have had longstanding fertility problems, miscarriages and/or children previously born with malformations or health problems, or where either prospective parent has had cancer, for a full house survey. We have found a number of houses where electromagnetism is present. People have then been able to re-position a bed or other much used piece of furniture, part with a DECT phone, or do whatever needed doing! Their health and ability to sleep has improved, and the following pregnancy has gone ahead successfully. As yet, information on this is not common knowledge, but I would not neglect this aspect of preconceptual care, as it is turning out to be a vital factor.

It is already standard practice that, apart from emergencies, medical X-rays are not used during pregnancy.

Further information on electromagnetic pollution and help in detecting and eliminating the sources can be obtained from:

Roy Riggs, 25 Coleridge Street, Hove, East Sussex, BN3 5AB. Tel: 01273 732523 www.royriggs.co.uk We have a DVD of Alfred Riggs and his work that you can hire for a week for £5.

Powerwatch U.K., Public Information, Borsham, Eccles, Suffolk, NR34 8HW Tel. Helpline £1.50 a minute 0897 100800 www.powerwatch.org.uk

OTHER HAZARDS

These constantly come to light, such as the toxic substances found in many household products, hair dyes, cosmetics and household cleaners. We suggest you use only natural and organic products wherever possible. See the list of Foresight publications for our "Watch It" booklet that gives more information about nasty chemical ingredients to avoid in cosmetics and toiletries.

We are threatened with having fluoride added to the tap water in more areas in the UK again, despite evidence that beneficial effects on children's teeth are minimal, and that it caused fluorosis (ugly patches on the front teeth), stomach upsets, porous bones, and more cases of cancer and leukaemia. Researchers in Florida also found it led to the birth of four times as many Down's Syndrome children. Avoid drinking treated water and using fluoride toothpaste, to minimise exposure. If you do live in an area where fluoride is already added we suggest that you have a water filter added to your tap that is capable of filtering out the fluoride from your drinking water (the Fresh Water Filter Company will be able to help you with this).

ULTRA-SOUND SCANS

Although now routinely used in pregnancy, there are suggestions that ultra-sound scanning can be dangerous, especially during the first three months of pregnancy, since during this time all the major parts of the baby are developing and are especially susceptible to malformations.

Further findings support the belief that ultra-sound has the capacity to damage unborn babies (BMJ, 3 & 17 July 1993)

> *"Though routine ultra-sound scanning does not improve the outcome of pregnancy, it exposes pregnant women to risk of false diagnosis of malformations, not to mention the possible brain damage".*   BMJ July 3rd 1993

Down the years we have noticed many people come to us after an in-utero death that occurred the same week as an early scan. AIMS, the Association for Improvements in Maternity Services, has made the same observation and they publish a little booklet "Ultrasound Unsound". We would advise reading this before making up your mind about whether or not to have the offered scans. Foresight advises avoiding scans unless they are considered essential for a specific reason.

You cannot be forced to have one, if you would rather not.

HOME BIRTHS

As the hazards of hospitalisation become greater – MRSA, and now PVL - Panton-Valentine Leukocidin, (a variant of MRSA) and Clostridium Difficile, quite apart from the risk of unnecessary intervention – the desirability and feasibility of home birth becomes greater. This is not our area of expertise, but while you are considering the venue for the birth, useful people to contact include:

The Royal College of Midwives, 15 Mansfield Street, London, W1G 9NH. (Tel: 020 7312 3535) www.rcm.org.uk

National Childbirth Trust (NCT) Alexandra House, Oldham Terrace, Acton, London, W3 6NH (Tel: 0870 444 8707) www.nct. org.uk

The Independent Midwives Association, 89 Green Lane, Farncombe, Surrey, GU7 3TB. (Tel: 0870 850 7539). www.independentmidwives.org.uk

SUMMARY

We suggest:
- Eating a diet along the Foresight Guidelines, filtering the water. A diet based on organic foods, unrefined carbohydrates, additive free. Plenty of organically reared protein foods. Plenty of raw fruit and vegetables.
- Obtaining Foresight hair analyses for help with a personalised vitamin and mineral programme.
- Avoiding smoking, alcohol, caffeine and street drugs completely, for both partners.
- Reviewing any use of medical drugs in the light of the intended pregnancy. (Involve your doctor, the drug manufacturer, and look on the web. Ask for written confirmation that it is safe in pregnancy.)
- Learning Natural Family Planning for use with abstention or the use of barriers during the six-day fertile phase.
- Checking out genito-urinary and other possibly hidden infections as well as Candida. Your local NHS Genito-Urinary Medicine Clinic will help you.
- Seeking help from a natural health practitioner if you need help with any health problems and including dealing with symptoms of stress. Neal's Yard Remedies have therapy rooms throughout the country with experienced practitioners.
- Seeking help where necessary with allergies, and/or intestinal parasites, and/or anorexic tendencies or obesity from a qualified practitioner.
- Being aware of possible electromagnetic pollution and seeking knowledgeable help.
- Joining Foresight and benefiting from the discounts on hair analysis and supplements, and regular news and views in the thrice-yearly newsletter.

FORESIGHT PUBLICATIONS

A stamped addressed envelope is appreciated

SUMMARIES

by Tuula Tuormaa - all 85p inc p&p

"The Adverse Effects of Manganese Deficiency on Reproduction".

"The Adverse Effects of Alcohol on Reproduction".

"The Adverse Effects of Tobacco Smoking on Reproduction".

"The Adverse Effects of Food Additives on Reproduction".

"The Adverse Effects of Genito-urinary Infection".

"The Adverse Effects of Zinc Deficiency"

"The Adverse Effects of Agrochemicals
        on Reproduction and Health".

"The Adverse Effects of Lead".

"The Role of Chromium, Selenium & Copper
        in Human and Animal Metabolism".

Chapter from "Vitamins in Endocrine Metabolism" by Isobel Jennings, 50p (plus 23p p&p)

POSTER

The full Foresight Programme £1.00 (plus £1.00 p&p).

CONTACTS

FORESIGHT
The Association for the Promotion of Pre-Conceptual Care,
178 Hawthorn Road, West Bognor, West Sussex PO21 2UY
Tel: 01243 868001
www.foresight-preconception.org.uk

WOMEN'S ENVIRONMENTAL NETWORK
PO Box 30626, London E1 1TZ
Tel: 0207 481 9004
www.wen.org.uk

NEAL'S YARD REMEDIES
• Therapy rooms with Foresight registered therapists
• Organic and natural skincare
• Herbs, supplements, homœopathic remedies and books.

To find your nearest shop or Therapy Rooms:
   telephone 01747 834634
   www.nealsyardremedies.com
   Mail order tel: 0845 262 3145